MW01222595

The Dash Diet Solution

Fast Weight Loss Guide

By Cathy Wilson
Copyright © 2014

Income Disclaimer

This book contains business strategies, marketing methods and other business advice that, regardless of my own results and experience, may not produce the same results (or any results) for you. I make absolutely no guarantee, expressed or implied, that by following the advice below you will make any money or improve current profits, as there are several factors and variables that come into play regarding any given business.

Primarily, results will depend on the nature of the product or business model, the conditions of the marketplace, the experience of the individual, and situations and elements that are beyond your control.

As with any business endeavor, you assume all risk related to investment and money based on your own discretion and at your own potential expense.

Liability Disclaimer

By reading this book, you assume all risks associated with using the advice given below, with a full understanding that you, solely, are responsible for anything that may occur as a result of putting this information into action in any way, and regardless of your interpretation of the advice.

You further agree that our company cannot be held responsible in any way for the success or failure of your business as a result of the information presented in this book. It is your responsibility to conduct your own due diligence regarding the safe and successful operation of your business if you intend to apply any of our information in any way to your business operations.

Terms of Use

You are given a non-transferable, "personal use" license to this book. You cannot distribute it or share it with other individuals.

Also, there are no resale rights or private label rights granted when purchasing this book. In other words, it's for your own personal use only.

The Dash Diet Solution

Fast Weight Loss Guide

By Cathy Wilson

Table of Contents

Introduction

As a qualified health and wellness expert, my aim is to open the door to finally reaching your fat loss, and health and wellness goals. This introductory guide will focus on uncovering the *ins* and *outs* of the world renowned Dash Diet, which according to the *US Department of Health and Human Services*, is the leading eating strategy with the purpose of halting deadly hypertension in its tracks.

I will remove all the unnecessary technical jargon, delivering take-action solutions that will guide and direct you towards your improved health and wellness goals, with renewed energy and strength.

KISS - Keep It Simple Stupid is what I've done.

FACT - What you choose to fill your belly with, when, and how much, directly affects every factor in your health. From obesity to diabetes, stroke and heart disease to motility and mobility issues, decision making, work performance, relationship issues, moods, your ability to perform in the bedroom, and even how long you'll live, are all reflective of your eating habits.

Your knowledge of food and commitment to make smart nutrition choices, determines in part, how much fat you're drop, whether or not it stays gone, and your overall picture of better health.

What unfortunately gets lost in the fog with these diet concepts, are all the other vital factors that have to

change in order for you to bask in the glory forever of optimal health!

What you don't know **WILL** hurt you.

It's time for positive change in your life. Make the decision to take control, open your mind to positive eating,
and other sustainable life changes that are going to make
you one sexy, hot, happy, and ridiculously healthy camp-
er, till death do you part.

Read on cuz you ARE worth it.

Chapter One - DASH DIET Basics

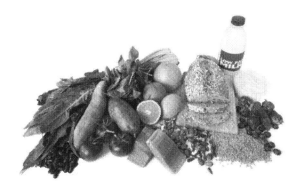

The Mayo Clinic, recognizes the DASH Diet, as emphasizing how much you're eating, and what you're eating, ensuring you're giving your body and mind a diverse range of healthy foods, that provide the nutrition you need to get, and stay healthy.

That's the nuts and bolts of the dash diet anyway.

So what does the DASH stand for?

Dietary Approaches to Stop Hypertension, which of course happens with wise-owl smart eating choices in moderation. So by testing the waters with this eating strategy, you're not only going to lower your blood pressure, but also reach out and positively touch all factors determining your health.

The state of your social, physical, mental, and environmental well-being, are dictated positively with healthier eating strategies. Which are ultimately attained through DASH Diet eating.

So why is this diet so popular?

It's versatile, sensible, doesn't use extreme measures, and can be adapted to just about any and all preferences and tolerances, if you set your mind to it.

In other words, it's doable long-term. A great place to start.

Who created this diet?

The National Lung, Blood, and Heart Institute.

Why should you test out this common sense eating strategy?

Other than the fact I said so! According to *WebMD*, once again, the DASH Diet was ranked best overall diet, from the *U.S. News & World Report*.

Often what creates resistance for many people looking to get skinny, is the lack of professional, and scientific validation behind a particular diet. The DASH Diet is an exception to the rules, cuz it's based on professional study and scientific evidence.

Up next, we'll have a look at the basics of how many calories your body needs, how to figure it out, and approximate food servings you'll require to reach your health and wellness goals.

My Thoughts...

Think of yourself as sitting in the pole position with this weight loss tool. There's no need to question whether it works or not, or if it's healthy for you on all levels. This diet has been pre-qualified, and passed with flying colors.

Now all you've got to do is learn your driving technique, so you can win your race to good health absolute!

Chapter Two - Basic Calories your Body Requires, How to Calculate, and Food Servings

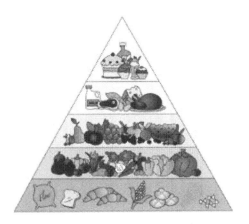

It makes zero sense for you to get all crazy excited about testing the waters with a new eating strategy, if you have no clue how many calories your body requires to thrive. This depends on your height and weight, gender, and activity level to start.

Of course, if we wanted to get technical, you go into your genetic makeup, the speed in which your body actually breaks down food, and even the actually timing of your tummy filling habits.

Basic is beautiful.

Here are a few pointers you need to understand, in order to lay the foundation for eating success.

Think *beginning,* and you're on the golden path.

BMI

In order to figure out how many calories your body needs to maintain your weight, you've gotta calculate approximately how many calories your body uses each day. If you're just focusing on healthier eating cuz your weight is just fine, then you can take a nap for a few minutes if you like.

The Dash Diet works based on a certain number of servings from each of the 8 food categories:

*Healthy Whole Grains
*Veggies
*Fruits
*Low-Fat Milk Products
*Lean Meat, Poultry, and Fish
*Legumes, Seeds, and Nuts
*Fats and Oils
*Added Sugars and Sweets

We are going to look at the average caloric needs of a woman with a moderate activity level, which is around 2200 calories/day to maintain weight.

This means, if this particular woman wants to lose weight, she's consistently going to have to take 500 calories off her bottom line per pound lost. This is best done with a combination of eating fewer overall calories, and exercising.

There are oodles of online calculators to help figure out your BMI. Otherwise your doctor, or fitness instructor can help you out. Math is not my strong suit, and I'm not afraid to say it!

According to the Dash Diet, a woman needing 2200 calories/day, would eat as follows...

6 servings Healthy Whole Grains
4-5 servings Veggies
4-5 servings Fruit
2-3 servings Low-Fat Milk Products
3-4 servings Lean Meat, Poultry, and Fish *Make note you need at least 2 servings fatty fish per week, to give your body a good dose of much needed omega-3 and 6 fatty acids!
2-3 servings healthy Fat/Oil
4 servings Nuts/Seeds/Legumes per week
5 or less servings Sweets and Added Sugar per week

Serving Sizes

This is the kicker when it comes to dropping flubber and getting healthy. So many people have no concept of what an actual true serving size is, what your body physiologically requires to function optimally.

I can guarantee, it's not **SUPER-SIZE**, and it certainly isn't even close to what a restaurant will slap down in front of you. Most restaurant servings are 2-3 times the portions your body actually needs.

Problem is, we've conditioned ourselves to **THINK** we need all that extra crap food, when the truth is nothing of the sort.

My Point - Serving sizes are heart function vital when committing to getting healthy for life, with the no-nonsense DASH Diet concept.

DASH Serving Suggestions

*Grains - 1 slice bread, 1/2 bagel, 3/4 cup cooked cereal, pasta, or rice, ounce of dry cereal

Food Examples - Whole grain bread, whole wheat bagel, brown rice, whole grain pasta, pita bread, English muffins, large flake oatmeal, grits, quinoa, air-popped popcorn, salt-free pretzels

Purpose - Provides long-term energy, essential vitamins and minerals, and fiber to help remove harmful toxins from your body.

*Veggies - 1 cup raw or steamed veggies, 1 cup leafy greens, 1/2 cup all-natural veggie juice

Food Examples - Carrots, kale, broccoli, spinach, turnip, peppers, sweet potato, beans, tomatoes (although technically a fruit), peas, celery,

Purpose - Loads of powerful protective antioxidants in brightly colored fruits, along with potassium, magnesium, and fiber.

*Fruits - 1 piece fruit, 1/2 cup fresh fruit, 1/4 cup dried fruit, 1/2 cup fresh fruit juice

Food Examples - Apples, oranges, grapefruit, bananas, pears, kiwi, starfruit, peaches, nectarines, grapes, cantaloupe, musk melon, watermelon, pineapple, raisins, strawberries, tangelos, tangerines, mangoes

Purpose - Offer antioxidant protection to deter free radicals from setting in, and creating disease, along with fiber, potassium, and magnesium.

*Low-Fat Milk Products - 1 cup low-fat milk, 3/4 cup yogurt, 2x2 inch cube cheese, 1/2 cup low-fat cottage cheese

Food Examples - Milk, yogurt, cottage cheese, hard cheese, fat-free frozen yogurt, low-fat rice pudding.

Purpose - Sources of calcium and protein to protect and strengthen bones and teeth, and to improve hair, skin, and nails.

*Lean Meat, Fish, Chicken, and Turkey - 1 ounce cooked meat or fish, 1 egg

Food Examples - Lean beef, skinless chicken and turkey, fish, shrimp, scallops, eggs

Purpose - Complete protein source to build strong muscles, provide energy, protein, magnesium, vitamins, and minerals.

*Legumes, Nuts, and Seeds - 1/3 cup nuts, 2 tablespoons seeds, 2 tablespoons peanut butter, 1/2 cup cooked legumes

Food Examples - Walnuts, almonds, peanuts, cashews, mixed nuts, sunflower seeds, sesame seeds, flax seeds, peanut butter, nut butter, kidney beans, chickpeas, lentils, peas

Purpose - Vital source of muscle building protein, fiber, energy, magnesium, and other essential vitamins, and minerals.

*Oil/Fat - 1 tsp oil, 1 tablespoon light mayonnaise, 2-3 tablespoon low-fat salad dressing

Food Examples - Olive, sunflower, almond, or vegetable oil, light mayonnaise, low-fat salad dressing, and Transfat free soft margarine.

Purpose - Fat is essential to survival, provides energy, insulates organs, joints, and tissues, and the brain is made primarily of fat. Without fat, you'd have a tough time thinking.

NOTE - The DASH Diet allots for about 27% fat from total calorie intake. It's a place to start, but definitely on the high end. Centres for Disease Control and Prevention states less than 10% of fat per day should come from saturated fats like butter, and animal fats. They suggest aiming for the lower end of the 20-30% of total daily calories from fat. Bottom line is, by eating a healthy balanced diet utilizing all the food groups, you'll have no worries giving your body the fat it requires to function optimally.

*Added Sugars/Sweets - 1/2 cup ice-cream, 1 tsp sugar, 2 tablespoons whipped topping, 1 tablespoon jam, 3/4 cup lemonade

Food Examples - Hard candy, ice-cream, syrup, sugar, sweet punch, gummy bears, jam, honey

My Thoughts...

Understanding how much food your body really needs, and what an actual serving size is, will help you gain the basics to bridge the gap between wanting and needing, learned unhealthy habits, and the creation of new better food choices.

With this base, you'll gain control of your weight, and overall health direction. You'll be back in the Captain's seat where you belong!

Just make sure you take the time to consciously acknowledge where you are right now on the health scale, and where you want to be. An important measurement factor to look back on one day with a gynormous smile.

COMMIT and you're good as gold in my books!

Chapter Three - Benefits DASH Diet

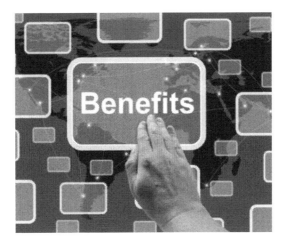

We already know the DASH Diet eating concept is based on eating less sodium to lower blood pressure.

Prevention and management are key.

The bottom line, is this long-term manageable eating plan improves your overall health by guiding you to make better food choices, or simply improve consistently day-to-day. A healthy route to getting healthy!

There's no...

*Starvation
*Forbidden Food Groups

*Restrictive Eating Times
*Complex Recipes
*Weighing Food
*Ordering Pre-Made Meals
*Fasting
*Food Boredom
*Extreme Measures

These are all factors that trigger diet failure.

The DASH Diet works. You can like it, or lump it.

This government recommended diet, based on fresh fruits and veggies, whole grain breads, low-fat milk products, and plant-based protein over meat, MAKES SENSE. It has impressive long-term benefits, like reducing the risk of stroke and cardiovascular disease, according to *PureHealthMD.*

We're going to have a gander a little later, on how salt reduction benefits your health. Just think of it as an upcoming feature.

Other Benefits of the Dash Diet Eating Strategy Are:

Easy to Follow - This diet is basic in nature. There are no specialty or pre-packaged foods you need to buy, which gets costly. It chooses healthy wholesome fruits and veggies, low-fat dairy products, and veggie protein sources first. The DASH Diet has staying power, because of the gynormous range of foods you can eat. One thing's for certain, you're never going to get bored!

Decreases Risk of Heart Disease and Stroke - According to *PureHealthMD*, a research study conducted over 25 years, on 25 year-old women, showed major health benefits with this diet. These subjects committed to eating a healthy diet of fruits, veggies, low-fat milk, and plant-based protein. The study concluded these women on the DASH Diet, were 24% less likely to have cardio-vascular disease, and 18% less likely to have a stroke, compared to women on the Standard American Diet.

*Lower Blood Pressure - Studies show individuals eating a diet high in fruits and veggies, and low-fat dairy, and lower in saturated fat, total fat, and cholesterol, had lower blood pressure.

The DASH Diet eating style is lower in salt and higher in calcium, potassium, fiber, and magnesium. It's this synergy created between nutrients that helps decrease blood pressure as much as some medications.

This is beneficial because the heart doesn't have to work as hard pumping nutrient-oxygen rich blood throughout your body. The arteries have more mobility too.

*Decreases Risk of Certain Cancers, Diabetes, Osteoporosis, and Kidney Failure - This eating concept has been coined a *diet for all diseases*, with benefits for everyone.

The...

-National Heart, Lung and Blood Institute
-American Heart Association
-Dietary Guidelines for Americans

ALL recommend the DASH Diet, because of the fantastic difference a few small eating changes can make.

My Thoughts...

25

Simple and tasty works for me! The DASH Diet takes you back to the basics. The natural evolutionary way humans were made to eat. Running from the learned unhealthy fast food, Trans fat, saturated fat loaded, processed food diet we've become accustom to.

You are what you eat, and the advantages of following the DASH eating strategy can't be ignored, not if you're serious about blasting fat, finding energy, deterring disease, controlling chronic pain, and flipping your frown upside down permanently!

Chapter Four - Limitations (red meat, sugar added, and fat added)

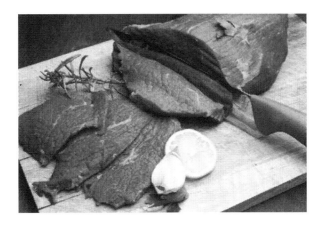

No *no-no's* of the DASH Diet eating concept, aside from excess sodium, are red meat, added sugars, and fat.

ASSUMPTIONS

I'm going out on a limb to say these are gynormous generalizations on the part of this diet, because there are a heck of a lot of assumptions being made. One, is that all these limitations are being over-consumed, which for the most part is likely correct, but not always.

Another, is the version eaten, is the *bad* one. So bad, saturated/Trans-fat versus good, unsaturated fat, for example. Brown and white sugar, instead of the natural sweetener in fruits, and the meat being chomped down is *fatty*.

Now these assumptions are true for the most part, considering the fact most people use the DASH Diet to blast flab, hopefully anyway, which means they are living an unhealthy lifestyle, or they wouldn't be porkers in the first place. That opens a whole new can of worms.

Although experts argue there are ways to include these DASH Diet *limitations*, in a healthy eating plan.

Why are people fat?

*Crap fast food/processed food eating
*Couch potatoes that play video games and are allergic to exercise
*Lack of mobility because of health issues, self-created, or plain bad luck
*Mental issues triggering overeating, a chemical imbalance making them fat, indirectly anyway
*The environment in which people live
*Stress
*Crappy social pressures
*Learned junky lifestyle

The only weakness I see with the DASH Diet, is there are oodles of assumptions. And that people may take the *limitations* of this diet too directly.

FACT: Red meat isn't BAD for you. But high fat red meat choices in excess are, along with red meat cooked in fat, in massive amounts.

A naked spinach salad with 1/2 cup of grilled lean beef **IS** healthy.

Sprinkling a teaspoon of sugar on a bowl of fresh berries **IS** healthier than adding 1/4 cup of sugar, or 1/2 cup whipping cream.

M-O-D-E-R-A-T-I-O-N

A teaspoon of butter on your veggies, is better than cook-ing them in oil, then added 1/4 cup butter.

Can you see where I'm going here?

Simply because people have such a diverse range of food knowledge in general, common sense, and ability to see balance in the big picture, diets often have to give everyone no candy, because some Yahoos will take and eat 100, instead of just one.

Something for you to think about with the DASH Diet, and all of your nutritional choices.

RED MEAT LIMITATION

Usually red meat is *off limits* in a heart healthy eating plan like the DASH Diet, because the gynormous leap focus is controlling unhealthy saturated fat. According to *Shape* magazine, both health professionals and social media has been mismanaging this message.

FACT: Low quality cuts of beef are high in saturated fat. But there are about 30 cuts of beef stamped lean by the USDA, with lower levels of saturated fat than chicken thighs!

Smart Red Meat Choices: Lean ground beef, shoulder pot roast, top round, flank steak, top loin, and T-bone steaks.

Store this information in you back pocket, just in case you're in a scenario where red meat is it. At least you'll have the ammo to choose wisely.

Did you know..._Penn State University_ conducted a study, following what 36 people put into their mouths for 6 months, and concluded lean ground beef is okay for the DASH Diet eating plan?

Reality - You can include 4 oz. of lean beef per day, and still fall within your daily allowance for saturated fat. Just be certain you watch the rest of your food choices carefully.

Extra Lean Meat - Has less than 5 grams of total fat, and less than 2 grams of saturated fat.

Lean Meat - Has less than 10 grams of total fat, and doesn't go higher than 4.5 grams of bad fat.

Cons Fatty Read Meat in the Extreme

*Some meats have high cholesterol and fat. This increases the risk of high cholesterol and cardiovascular disease.

*Conventionally raised beef is pumped with antibiotics, and hormones. Which is incredibly difficult to measure the impact with human consumption, but it is negative. Many healthcare professionals believe it's linked to cancers, and various other serious disease.

*Don't forget about the pesticides and chemicals the animals were exposed to growing up. These harmful substances filtrate into the meat you eat.

Sample High Fat Meat: (fat per 3-ounce serving)

-Regular ground beef - 230 calories - 15 g total fat - 5.7 saturated fat

-Beef ribs - 200 calories - 11 g total fat - 4.5 g saturated fat

-Beef brisket - 185 calories - 8.6 g total fat - 3.1 g saturated fat

-Medium ground beef - 180 calories - 10 g total fat - 4 g saturated fat

-Porterhouse steak - 180 calories - 9.4 g total fat - 3 g saturated fat

Saturated Fat - Saturated fats have been around since the beginning of civilization. However in the past 75 years, societal health has taken a turn for the worst, and unhealthy saturated fats are a key contributor.

Our modern day lifestyles, eating habits, and exposure to toxins, have definitely triggered serious disease, including heart disease.

The proof is in the pudding, as our ancestors certainly didn't face the degree of chronic health issues we battle today.

Facts Saturated Fat:

*Fats that have carbon bonds full
*Solid at room temperature
*Linked to serious disease like heart disease, Alzheimer's, diabetes, and cancer

NOTE- When healthy polyunsaturated fats are exposed to oxygen, they turn from a liquid to semi-solid, and eventually turn rancid. This often happens when these once-upon-a-time good fats, spend too much time in a ware house, and turn bad. This fat is more dangerous than saturated fats. Funny how this issue never seems to make it to the front page.

ADDED SUGAR LIMITATION

Are you someone that adds sugar to sweeten your strawberries, cereal, or morning beverage?

A learned habit that often escalates over time. From a sprinkle to a teaspoon, to a 1/4 cup, without consciously recognizing it, happens fast. Experts at *Care2*, report added sugar triggers cell inflammation. Way down deep inside your body, the tiny cuts made by the sugar, continue to fester silently. It's not noticeable, because this destructive process evolves just below the height of your pain threshold.

Clever how much control your mind and body have naturally.

Over time, added sugar causes serious health issues, because of the repetitive cellular damage.

Think of it like you would blowing up a balloon. Eventually it's going to bust wide open. That's when suddenly, a life-threatening disease smacks you square in the face.

Some of these disease are:

*Cancer - Cancerous cells are addicted to glucose. In fact, when a patient is scanned for cancer, they drink a sugary solution, and doctors observe possible malignancies that suck up the sugars.

32

Dr. Don Ayer, of the Huntsman Cancer Institute in Salt Lake City, says if you can restrict glucose metabolism, you can stop cancer growth.

A bold but promising statement.

*Heart Disease - Studies published in the *American Medical Association,* showed people getting 25% or more of their daily calories from added sugar, gynormously increased their risk for high cholesterol, and unhealthy levels of blood fats, or triglycerides. Both of which are causal factors for heart disease.

The DASH Diet deters heart disease, by making sure added sugars are avoided. A mind over matter issue when it's consciously recognized. The problem arises when sugars are cleverly hidden in foods. One matter-of-fact reason to steer clear of processed foods!

*Type 2 Diabetes - For the most part, type 2 diabetes is preventable. Poor eating, little exercise, and crap lifestyle habits, increase the risk gynormously. This deadly disease causes blindness, nerve damage, the amputation of limbs, and is hands down the most direct and deadly consequence of excess sugar.

Nearly 25 million Americans have been diagnosed. It's a number that continues to climb at an alarming rate.

Essentially what happens, is your cells stop responding to insulin, and glucose builds up in the blood because your cells can't absorb it. This triggers inflammatory health issues.
Another problem, is that before diabetes is actually diagnosed, metabolic syndrome (inflammation), issues war

on your body, triggering heart disease and cancer, among others.

One in-your-face reason **PREVENTION** is critical, which is exactly what the DASH Diet represents.

Your golden ticket to prevention!

*Immune System Weakness - Too much sugar causes biochemical stress on your system, along with inflammation, which causes too much stress on the body, and weakens your immune system function.

Too much sugar causes leaky gut. This is where unprocessed food molecules get into your blood, and your immune system has to work double shifts, digesting the food in your bloodstream too. In time, your immune system gets worn out and doesn't respond. Then you're in oodles of trouble.

Psoriasis, lupus, and arthritis, are all indicators of an immune system that's working way too hard.

*Yeast Infections - Candida, or yeast infections, are a fungal infection. What you eat can influence your risk. According to doctors at *The Mayo Clinic*, blood sugar levels are directly linked to these itchy infections. If you have diabetes, your risk increases for getting the infection.

It's recommended you eat a healthy diet, like the DASH Diet, to balance hormones and regulate good health.

And although medical research hasn't confirmed it yet, experts believe too much sugar, combined with stress, triggers yeast infections.

That's all I need to know!

FAT LIMITATION - Not only does the DASH Diet limit salt and cholesterol intake, but also bad fat.

Fat Facts

You can't live without fat. Your body can't produce EFAs, essential fatty acids without fat, according to *Dr. Wahida Karmally* of Columbia University.

Fat transports the fat-soluble vitamins A, D, E, and K, in and around your body, via your blood.

Good fat is essential for brain development, eyesight, and healthy skin and hair development.

*Fat has more than **TWICE** the calories of protein or car-bohydrates.*

*Two much fat increases risk of heart and stroke.

Fat in excess will clog arteries, and block adequate oxy-gen stores from reaching your heart and brain.

20-30% of your diet should come from healthy fats, ac-cording to The American Heath Association. Unfortunately, American's get more than **THIRTY-FOUR** percent. That's where the DASH Diet eating strategy swoops in and saves the day!

By following the DASH Diet, you'll eat a balanced diet full of fresh fruits and veggies, lean milk products, and plant-based protein sources, that minimizes fat consumption without getting technical, and reduces your risk for serious disease, while gaining energy, and losing weight.

My Thoughts...

When it comes to eating or diet limitations, it's critical to look at both sides of the coin. Anything to the extreme isn't a good move. What you need to understand, is that eating in excess with any type of food, protein, carbs, or fat, can make you fat!

The DASH Diet limitations in salt, added sugars, excess fat, and red meat, are benchmarks or red flags, to set you up for success in your eating habits. As you learn to adapt your new healthy eating habits through DASH eating, you'll have the knowledge to decide what food limitations work for you, and which ones don't.

Finding your eating style is a learning process, with prerequite courses on handling a heck of a lot of trial and error.

*You are wise-owl smart to start the DASH Diet eating concept, as per the rules with limitations. After you've earned your degree, you've got the physiological means to tinker with the rules a little. Understanding nothing is written in stone. The goal is to figure out the best eating changes **you** can make, that will stick forever!*

*The DASH Diet **WILL** help.*

Chapter Five - Ultimate KEY Factor DASH DIET – SALT

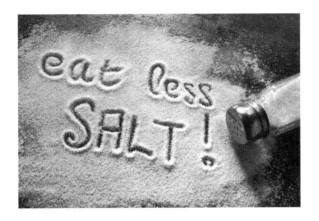

Where do we get most of our added salt from?

CRAPPY processed fast food eating. It's convenient, cheap, and downright addictive. Not to mention it plays nicely into the emotional roller coaster lives we live.

PROBLEM - Too much salt.

SOLUTION - Eating healthy, all-natural foods found in the DASH Diet. Combined with regular exercise your body has intrinsically required physiologically, since before you took your first breath!

You eat processed foods loaded with salt. Sprinkle it on your veggies, potato, and pretty much any dish set in front of you. It's habitual for most. A nasty bad habit you don't really need physically or mentally, but do anyway.

Unconscious habits for many eventually **KILL**.

By conditioning your body to expect this naturally occurring mineral, you're just going to keep on sprinkling it on until you get slapped in the face with serious disease.

PREVENTION is critical, and the DASH Diet brings sodium to your attention, giving you the platform to take action.

Why do you need Salt?

Your body can't function without salt. It's essential for optimal nervous system function. However, a balance in required to recognize the benefits of salt, and deter serious health consequences from arising with too much.

You need salt for...

Membrane Function - Sodium, chloride, and potassium, are necessary for keeping your electrochemical balance between the environment within your cells, and the surrounding fluid, referred to as the membrane potential.

Sodium helps regulate nerve impulses and muscle contractions.

Blood Volume - Sodium helps maintain blood volume. Your body needs a certain level of salt in the blood. When you eat too much salt, your body is forced to retain water to help dilute the salt in your blood.

To sum up, you need sodium to...

-Maintain fluid levels
-Transmit nerve impulses

-Optimal muscle contraction and relaxation

How much salt do you need?

*One teaspoon of table salt, sodium and chloride, equates to 2300 mg of sodium.

The Dietary Guidelines for Americans suggest no more than 2300 mg of sodium each day. Less if you are over the age of 50, have diabetes, high blood pressure, kidney disease, or are black.

Best mindset...less is more.

The DASH Diet focuses on proper amounts of healthy eating, to reduce overall sodium intake to healthy levels. By eating foods with less salt than the basic American diet, you'll decrease your total salt intake, which triggers high blood pressure, and serious disease from there.

The DASH Diet allows for 2300mg of salt per day, but encourages 1500 mg, to see more dramatic results.

Did you know?

The typical American diet takes in between 3500 and 5000 mg of sodium per day!

Consequences of Too Much Sodium

Too much sodium over time has serious ramifications

*High Blood Pressure

Too much salt triggers water retention, promoting issues with the influx of water into your blood vessels. This shocks your blood pressure to rise, by increasing your blood volume, and constricting flow.

Hypertension triggers serious deadly diseases, like heart disease and stroke.

*Kidney Issues

Too much salt filtrates through to your urine. This strains the natural filtration process of your kidneys, increasing crystallization.

*Heart Issues

Eating too much salt makes your heart work harder. Over time this can lead to an enlarged heart, which means your heart is weakened and prone to malfunctioning more often than a healthy heart.

*Osteoporosis

Studies show salt interferes with calcium absorption. Bottom line is, if you're eating too much salt in your diet, your bones will suffer.

*Gastrointestinal Diseases

Your blood acid-base balance is dependent on sodium. Too much will cause acid reflux, which causes long-term damage to your digestive system. Research shows too much salt is a strong factor for some cancers, ulcers, and gut issues.

*Swelling/Dehydration

Drinking salt makes you thirsty, because the salt draws water out of your sells and into your body tissues. Just think bloating and you're on track!

Less salt reduces swelling.

*Hormonal Imbalance

Too much salt interferes with the chemical balance in your body. This can trigger cramping, dizziness, and shaking.

EVIL SALTY FOODS

Soya Sauce - 2300 mg per teaspoon

Other High Salt Sauces and Dressings - Teriyaki, steak sauce, barbecue sauce

Roquefort Cheese - 507 mg per ounce

Other High Salt Sauces and Dressings - Romano, Blue Cheese, Parmesan

Cooked Meat - Bacon - 170 mg per slice

Other High Salt Cured Meats - Cod, anchovy, beef jerky, smoked salmon, salami

Packaged Soup - 750 mg per pouch

Pickles - 750 mg per pickle

Fast Food Ham and Egg Biscuit - 1000 mg per serving

Other High Salt Fast Foods - Burritos, fries, chicken sandwich, burger, pizza, hash browns

Salted Nuts - 700 mg per ounce

Canned Veggies - 1000 mg per half cup

Junk Snacks - Pretzels - 450 mg per ounce

Other High Salt Snacks - Chips, microwave popcorn, theater popcorn, taco chips, crackers

BETTER FOOD CHOICES (According to Health-LinkBC - Less than 120 mg/serving)

Milk Products - Milk, unsalted cheese, yogurt, soy beverage

Healthy Whole Grains - Rice, quinoa, barley, oats, pasta, noodles, unsalted crackers and breadsticks, breadcrumbs, banana bread, muffins, cornbread, rice

Meat and Meat Alternates - Meat, turkey, chicken, fish, shellfish, low salt canned fish, eggs, unsalted nuts, seeds, and butter, lentils, tofu

Veggies and Fruit - All veggies and fruits, low salt canned veggies, tomato paste, low sodium fruit and veggie juices

Soups - Low sodium soup or cubes, homemade soup with no salt added

Fats - Butter, margarine, and unsalted sauces and salad dressings

Pointers to Lower Sodium

*Naturally decrease salt intake, and your body will adjust

*Eat more whole foods, and less processed

*Take restaurant cooking home, with less salt

*Choose lean meats with low sodium

*Flavor food with herbs and spices, not salt

*Buy low-sodium versions

*Check the nutrition label in packaged foods

*Stop and taste **BEFORE** you shake

My Thoughts...

Sodium is a love-hate relationship. You need it to live, but it will kill you if you abuse it. Finding your balance of sodium through the strategies of the DASH Diet, will only improve your health, mentally, and physically.

Change is tough, but if you commit to start taking the obvious added salt out of your eating, and then battle the hidden stashes, your kidneys, mind, and body, will thank you for it!

*One step at a time. One manageable change at a time, and you **WILL** make a difference!*

Chapter Six - Weight Loss and DASH

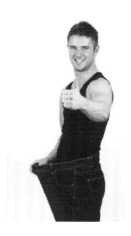

FACT: According for *Disease Control and Prevention*, 78 million Americans, or 1/3 of the population are obese.

FACT: Main diseases related to obesity are stroke, heart disease, cancer, and diabetes, all leading causes of preventable death.

FACT: Obese individuals in America cost over 150 billion dollars in medical costs yearly. Obese people cost over $1500 more per year than normal weight individuals.

The DASH Diet supports sustainable healthy fat loss.

Plan to lose weight includes:

*Oodles of fruits and veggies that are high fiber, and low calories.

*Moderate exercise is recommended, which supports weight loss, better than a sharp stick in the eye! However, I feel you've everything to gain by incorporating an intense kick-ass interval training regimen daily.

Go big or go home. Reach for the stars, and if you get halfway there, you've succeeded!

*Meals and snacks include lean healthy proteins, dense in nutrients to keep your hunger satiated longer, and your energy levels flying high and level. No crashing allowed!

*Your mindset is trained positive. Focus on the healthy new foods you're creating into habit, and you won't have time to cry a river over the crap foods you're letting go.

*Till death do you part is the focus. So if you're looking for a short-term relationship, get lost!

*Good carbs are kept under control to promote longer term energy. Starches are limited. Protein is readily available to build and support muscle, provide energy, and keep your metabolism flying high.

This plan is flexible, and promotes fast healthy weight loss with smart, versatile, and diverse eating.

BENEFITS OF LOSING WEIGHT

Work Advantage - Behavioral therapist *Robinson Welch*, PhD, says when eating out with co-workers, if you eat healthy, your boss and co-workers will notice. This

can go a heck of a long way when it's time for a job pro-
motion.

*Nicer to your Wallet - Prevention reports, slashing just
100 calories a day will save you about 200 bucks in food
per year. Sounds like a deal to me!

*Get your Sex Back! - Research shows, men with an
extra 30 pounds on them, have testosterone levels similar to men 10 years older.

*Social Butterfly Status - Popularity increases the more
fit/active you are.

*Avoiding Diabetes - Obesity increases the risk of insulin malfunction, and diabetes developing. When you're
fat, your cells have a difficult time responding to insulin.
This makes internal systems work harder, and diabetes
may become your reality.

Studies show, that losing as little as 10% of your body
weight can decrease your diabetes risk by almost 60%!
The DASH Diet is a fantabulous place to start.

*Better Blood Glucose Levels - By getting your weight
in the normal range, you'll have better control of your
blood glucose levels, which influence mood, energy levels, and temperament, along with offsetting some of the
complications of diabetes, including kidney failure, blindness, stroke, heart disease, and amputations.

***Lowers Cholesterol and Risk for Heart Disease and
Stroke** - The two main risks for heart disease are elevat-
ed cholesterol and blood pressure. *The American
College of Cardiology,* states too much body fat creates
and releases chemicals into your bloodstream that trig-

gers a rise in blood pressure, forcing the liver to make more bad (LDL) cholesterol.

Makes sense as you lose weight, the blood pressure drops down, and your liver reduces the LDL production.

Better Sleep - Fat people tend to have more soft tissue in the neck area, often obstructing breathing and causing snoring. This interferes with quality sleep. Snoring may also be a symptom of a life-threatening condition called sleep apnea, where breathing actually stops up to 50 times an hour in serious cases!

This forces the individual to wake up repeatedly, again, making a quality uninterrupted 7-8 hour sleep impossible. This oxygen deprivation has serious consequences over time. Including sex issues, concentration and memory problems, heart problems, and immunity issues.

Experts at **healthyweightforlife.com** report, even a 10% weight loss reduces snoring, and the number of sleep apnea episodes per night by up to 30%.

Improved Mobility and Motility - The heavier you are, the harder your body has to work physically to move. Remove your 25 pound back pack, and instead of huffing and puffing up the stairs, you'll fly! Losing weight will also enable you to reach where you've never reached before!

Increased Energy - The physiological benefits of losing weight, eating healthy, exercising, and maintaining your weight are gynormous. Increased self-esteem, optimism, energy, and lower rates of depression and chronic disease, are associated scientifically with flab loss.

Improved Fertility - Although the scientific community has yet to find concrete evidence, they've observed a relationship between obesity and fertility, and confirm it interferes with making babies. Exactly how or why is still foggy. But the experts guess is that fat interferes with sex hormone balance, and the actual ability for an obese woman to ovulate.

If she isn't releasing an egg, making a baby isn't going to happen. Some women even have bleeding similar to a period, where they think they've ovulated, but haven't. This is called an ovulatory cycle.

Being overweight during pregnancy also increases the risk from complications. Gestational diabetes, sleep apnea, forced caesarean delivery, huge babies, hard labour, and birth-related deaths, all increase in obese mothers.

Losing weight increases the chances of getting knocked up, and decrease the risks for trouble throughout the pregnancy term.

*Strengthened Immune System - Losing weight enables your body to function more efficiently as a whole. Your system is less sluggish, and your internal circuits are humming nicely. This ensures your immune system has the ammo it needs to battle free radicals looking to take you down by creating disease.

Losing weight will also lift your spirits, which research has shown, reduces the number of illness bouts you'll face.

*Increased Optimism - When you're losing weight, looking good and feeling fantabulous, that's gotta boost self-esteem and life optimism. We are a society driven by materialism, always wanting bigger, stronger, faster, thinner, and better.

Skinny is in your face 24/7. The magazines and television shows remind you of this, along with family and friends sometimes.

Psychologist *Leland Cliver*, states that health changes for the better, including weight loss, trigger positive emotion, which makes the good better, and the rotten, not so bad.

Increased optimism walks hand in hand with fat loss.

My Thoughts...

The DASH Diet promotes healthy weight loss. The above benefits are just the tip of the iceberg. The longer you commit to eating healthy, and the more pounds you drop, the greater the rewards; mentally and physically.

You are important.
Your health and life are important.
Time for you to make eating changes for the better, one manageable step at a time.

Chapter Seven - VIP Factors Optimal Health

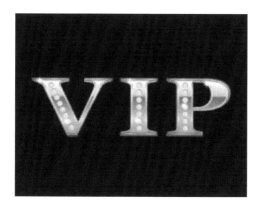

According to *WHO, World Health Organization,* there are numerous factors that determine the health of an individual. Yes, how you fuel your body, when, and how much is a vital piece of the multifactorial puzzle of good health.

However, there's oodles more to it.

Unfortunately, most diet plans fall short in communicating clearly. You've gotta do a heck of a lot more than choose whole wheat over white, pick lean beef over a greasy burger, and toss your chips for a bowl of fresh fruit, to gain optimal health.

The *World Health Organization* defines health as, **"a state of complete physical, mental, and social well-being and not merely the absence of disease or infirmity."**

This encompasses a heck of a lot more than just the DASH Diet, or any other eating strategy for that matter.

What you eat is critical in good health, but so are these factors:

***Social and Economic Environment** - The people you hang around, your social status, family support and attitude, education, job status, and access to health services, are just a few factors that are considerate of good health.

Some of these factors are controllable, and others aren't so cut and dry. You only know what you know, and your environment influences your character and life decisions. If you happen to grow up in a negative family environment, where nobody exercises, fast food IS the menu, and nothing you do is ever right, you're at a disadvantage when it comes to good health, because you haven't been taught the basics, you didn't ever learn to pay attention to your health and happiness.

Your social circle is gynormously reflective of your health. It's really tough to get healthy when all of your friends are overweight, junky eating gamers that consider sweating for anything a punishment.

As humans, we are intrinsically or genetically programmed to want to fit in. Everyone wants to feel needed, loved, and respected. Even the bad-asses!

Maslow's Social Needs Hierarchy, talks about love, acceptance, and belonging. Where humans need:

*Friends
*Romantic relations

*Family
*Social groups
*Religious organizations
*Community relations

All necessary to ward off loneliness, and more serious mental illnesses like depression and anxiety.

If you aren't happy in your environment and social relations as a whole, chances are your self-worth will suffer. Negative feelings, in general, increase the chances you're not going to care about yourself. You will play into how you're feeling by eating crappy simple sugar high calorie fatty foods, and not committing to any sort of exercise regimen, because you don't have the energy, want, or desire.

Health issues that arise are also less likely to get the attention they deserve because you're feeling hopeless, and *think* you really don't care.

In order to get healthy, you've gotta get your social and environmental status positive.

Quick Tip Action Steps to Improve Your Social

Listen - People want to be heard, and learning to listen improves your like-ability factor gynormously.

Try a New Hobby - A great way to make new friends and social connections, is open your mind to newness, and experience new things. Discovering a new hobby is exciting, and finding new people to share it with is even better.

Random Acts of Kindness - I believe in this one whole heartedly. Just think of how good it feels to make someone smile. It's the simple things that matter. Shovelling the neighbors' driveway, paying for a random strangers' coffee, or how about taking someone to a doctors' appointment because you can.

Small gestures that are a win-win every time.

Turn off the Bloody Phone! - It's great to be connected. But give yourself permission to turn your phone off and interact with the people around you. Physical face 2 face communication is slowly, but surely, fading away in our society. And the physical is something you need to find your balance.

Do yourself a favor and shut off your devices, and learn to communicate with your species.

Learn Empathy - Everyone has a story. By making the time to empathize and try to understand what people are going through, you're going to establish that much needed trust factor with people, which of course increases your social well-being.

Make a Point of Saying "I Love You." - This is probably the most powerful phrase we have. One that you'll never be sorry you said, but will regret it if you don't. Make a habit of it, and you'll strengthen your social.

Take Action and Create Happiness - Research shows people that take the initiative to optimistically take life by the horns, repeatedly have stronger social relations, than individuals that sit back and watch life pass them by.

Your reality is what you make it.

I believe this with every fiber of my being.

Focus on People - When someone is talking to you, make sure you warrant them your undivided attention. This means your eyes aren't wandering around the room checking out all the hotties, and you're not checking e-mails and texts.

Manners are important. Make a point of giving people your attention, and you'll seek favoritism in the social department.

Don't be Gun Shy - Don't be afraid to approach people to strike up a conversation. When you're in line at the coffee shop, talk to the Yahoo standing beside you. Ask them how there day's going, or perhaps even talk about the weather if you're that desperate.

Learn to Give Compliments - People love to get compliments. Just makes their day a tad bit brighter. If you like the sexy leather jacket the young man sitting near you is wearing, TELL HIM! Perhaps you love the color of the cashier's nails. Don't be afraid to say so.

Making a routine of giving compliments to people, is going to make both of you feel fantastic. Socially this is a wise-owl move.

*Physical - According to *Dr. Travis Saunders*, regular physical exercise will add years of quality life to your agenda. This should be enough to cohere your butt up off the couch and into action!

Here are a Few Simple Routes to Get Your Physical On!

Park your Car a Few Blocks Away - Making a habit of parking your car a few blocks away from you destination, is going to start the ball rolling getting physical exercise into your day. The first step is the biggest!

Turn your television off and go outside - Unfortunately, television watching has turned into a learned obsession for many people. The great news is, it can be unlearned too!
Make a point of turning off the television so you can find some other active way to occupy your time. Maybe you want to take a walk around the block. Start cleaning up your yard. Or perhaps even hopping on your rustic bike and going for a spin.

Doesn't really matter what you do, as long as you get your heart rate up! And yes, this includes having sex!

CHALLENGE YOURSELF! - Make a game of consciously putting more effort into every physical thing you do. So when you're vacuuming, pick up the pace. If you're hiking up and down the stairs a zillion times a day, do it faster. Even when you're scooting to the car, try and do it in at a runner's pace. The ideas is to put a little controlled effort into maximizing the energy you burn, with every move you make.

A little eventually adds up to gynormous!

Physical Transportation - It's understandable there are going to be times where riding your bike isn't going to work, not to mention it could even be illegal if you've got to take highways to get there. But you can choose to walk, take public transportation, or ride your bike on occasion. All of which is going to get your body moving, if you commit to making the move challenging.

Hit the Gym at Lunch or Take a Walk - A fantabulous way to get exercise into your busy day is to use your work break or lunch time to hit the gym, or even scoot out for a brisk walk. Getting some intense interval training in at the gym, lifting weights, and challenging your heart, are fantabulous routes to getting your mental and physical set to handle the rest of the day.

You'll kick into your endorphins, leaving you feeling energetic, optimistic, alive, and rarin' to go.

Don't make excuses. Try it - You'll LOVE it!

Set Yourself up for Success - Finding an activity you love to do, is only going to increase the odds you're going to make your new physical activities stick for the long run. There's no use taking an aerobics class, if you hate group things, or try a class during the wee hours of the morning when you're a night hawk, and don't really have the money to spare for it.

There are ten zillion different things you can do to get physically healthy. Join a gym with a trainer, ride your bike and lift weights at home, join a biking or running club, or maybe even sign yourself up for rigorous salsa dancing.

Where there's a will there's a way!

Shout it out to the World - Having supports in place to encourage you to stick to your game plan is golden. Find a workout partner, or make sure your friends ask you about your new biking group.

It seems easy for us to disappoint ourselves, but a lot tougher when we're letting others down too.

Emotional/Mental - *familydoctor.org* recognizes stress plays a pivotal role in your emotional or mental well-being, which is directly linked to good health. Finding your balance emotionally, is going to help you better cope with life challenges.

It's not so much the issues you face, but how you handle them that matters.

Here are a Few Basic Tips to Get You Mentally Happy!

Take Regular Timeouts - By making the time to calm your mind and body regularly, you're going to set yourself up for mental balance. Meditation and yoga are great habits to create. It can also be as simple as taking a quiet walk, or maybe a nice warm bubble bath.

Make some time to chill each day, and your mind will thank you for it!

Make Time to do Things you enjoy - People get happy when they're doing things they love. If you like hiking, make the time to fit it into your schedule regularly. If shopping is your cup of tea, get at least a couple cups each week. Maybe you've got a favorite movie you love. So find some time to watch it.

You know you, or at least I hope you do. Consider your preferences and tolerances, and opt to do the things you love.

Take Care of Your Health - Once it's gone, it's gone! Your health is the most valuable asset you own. Unfortunately, we spend a life-time abusing our shell. We make poor eating choices, don't bother exercising, forget how to vent our frustrations, and create the stressful life in which we live.

You've gotta take care of you! This means making a point of eating right on the DASH Diet. Incorporate exercise into your daily regimen, and make sure you find time to get your head on straight.

You should go to the doctor regularly, visit the dentist to make sure your smile is healthy, and schedule regular visits to the gym and your yoga sessions, because you deserve to be healthy and happy!

This should be reason enough to **take action** and just do it!

*Personal Characteristics and Learned Behaviors - Your personal characteristics and learned behaviors are reflective of your good health. Many develop over time. Some are learned, others are controllable, or not.

According to *Harvard Medical*, experts believe long-term change happens when it's self-rooted and based on positive thought. In other words, if you're trying to lose weight because your partner said you were fat, and not because you *want* to, it's not going to happen. Or at least it won't stick for the long run.

Being motivated by guilt, fear, or regret, all negative emotions, isn't healthy.

Here are a Few Pointers to Help You Establish Positive Change That Sticks!

Make Goals Specific - When you're not overwhelming yourself with too much change, the odds of succeeding increases gynormously. Define your positive behavioral changes specifically. For example, aim to get your butt into bed by 11 pm EVERY night, so you get the sleep your body needs to perform optimally. Make sure you plan your meals, so you're not binge eating cause your emotions interfere with logic when you're tired and grumpy, and your tummy's rumblin'.

Set small manageable changes and you WILL succeed.

Commit When Mentally Ready - We're all guilty of this one. How many times have you said you're going to start eating healthy, only to throw in the towel the first night out with friends? Or how about joining the gym as your New Year's resolution, only to fade off into the sunset a few weeks later?

You've got to figure out that your health is important to you, and commit your mind to accepting this and taking action.

The only person you control is YOU!

Practice Repetition - The only way to create a new healthy habit is to repeat often. Research shows it takes up to 6 months of repeating a new action, to transform it into habit, where you don't need to focus your mental on it, cuz your mind and body know what to do.

Don't Focus on the Negative Behavior - The most effective route to weed out the negative behaviors in your life, is to add positive ones. If you are focusing on the negative, they will interfere with your passion to move forward positively. Instead, keep your positive actions center stage, and eventually the crap will dissipate and be forgotten.

Accept Setbacks - According to *Prevention* magazine, every effort you make in the right direction is worthwhile. It's inevitable there will be setbacks when setting your mind to make change. Deal with them as they come, and never let them steer you off course and into oncoming traffic.

Think of them as a bump in the road that eventually goes by the wayside.

Your thoughts and beliefs are your reality.

My Thoughts...

Your physical, mental, and social, are all key players in the big picture game of great health. The DASH Diet is a fantabulous eating platform concept from which to build your healthy nutrition base. Add to that intense regularly interval training, including strength training, stretching, weights, and cardio, along with strong social connections, and time for yourself to climb towards mental balance, and you've got a fantastic plan to get healthy; mind, body, and soul.

Great health is something you commit to bettering every day, in all areas. It's not something you get to pick and choose in, or something that stops and starts when you see fit.

You owe it to yourself to make the choice to start working towards good health. And the DASH Diet, is a wise-owl place to start!

Chapter Eight - Sample Eating Dash Diet

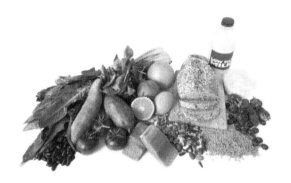

The DASH DIET...

*Limits sodium to 1500 - 2300 mg per day
*Rich in fruits, veggies, grains, low-fat dairy
*Limits total fat and cholesterol
*High fiber, potassium, calcium, and magnesium

Here's the recommended DASH Diet servings and serving sizes for the average woman that's moderately active, requiring 2000 calories a day:

Healthy Whole Grains

6-8 servings per day
Example Serving Size - 1/2 bagel, 1 slice bread, 1/2 cook cereal, 1/2 rice or pasta

Vegetables

4-5 servings per day
Example Serving Size - 1 cup leafy green veggies, 1/2 cooked veggies, 1/2 cup veggie juice

Fruits

4-5 servings per day
Example Serving Size - 1 piece fruit, 1/2 cup fresh or frozen fruit, 1/2 cup natural fruit juice, 1/4 cup dried fruit

Low-Fat Milk Products

2-3 servings per day
Example Serving Size - 1 cup milk, 1 oz. hard cheese, 1 cup yogurt

Lean Meat, Chicken, Turkey, and Fish

6 or less servings per day
Example Serving Size - 2 egg whites, 1 egg (limit to 3-4 per week), 1 oz. skinless poultry/lean meat/fish

Nuts, Seeds, and Legumes

4-5 servings per week
Example Serving Size - 2 tbsp. peanut butter, 1/3 cup mixed nuts, 2 tbsp. seeds, 1/2 cup legumes

Fats and Oils

2-3 servings per day
Example Serving Size - 1 tsp veggie oil, 1 tbsp. mayo, 2 tbsp. salad dressing, 1 tsp soft margarine

Sweets/Added Sugars

5 servings or less per week
Example Serving Size - 1 tbsp. jelly or sugar, 1/2 cup
sorbet, 1 cup lemonade

SAMPLE MEAL PLANS

Sample Day 1

Breakfast

1 slices whole grain toast with 2 tablespoons natural
peanut butter
1 orange
1 serving yogurt
Decaf coffee
Water

Lunch

Spinach salad
  *3 cups spinach
  *1 sliced apple
  *1/2 orange sliced
  *2 tbsp. crushed cashews
  *2 tbsp. low-fat salad dressing
6 wheat crackers
1 cup milk

Dinner

3 ounces grilled smoked salmon
1/2 cup whole grain pasta
1/2 cup asparagus
1 small whole wheat bun
1 cup fruit cup

Tea
Water

Snacks (anytime)

3/4 cup low-fat cottage cheese
4 arrowroot crackers

Nutrition Analysis

Calories - 1700
Cholesterol - 60 mg
Protein - 85 g
Sodium - 1500 mg
Carbs - 240 g
Fiber - 45 g
Total fat - 50 g
Potassium - 3300 mg
Saturated fat - 6 g
Calcium - 1200 mg

Sample Day 2

Breakfast

1 cup yogurt
1 cup mixed berries
1 small whole grain bran muffin
1 cup milk
Tea
Water

Lunch

Grilled chicken wrap
  *1 whole grain wrap
  *1/2 cup grilled chicken

*1/2 cup chopped pear
 *2 tbsp. low-fat mayo
  1 cup raw celery/carrots
  1 cup milk

Dinner

1 cup cooked quinoa
1 cup sliced tomato
2 cups leafy greens
1 tbsp. fat-free dressing
1 whole grain roll
1 clementine
Water

Snacks (anytime)

1/4 cup raisins, 25 unsalted pretzels, 1 tbsp. pumpkins
seeds, 1 tbsp. sunflower seeds

Nutrition Analysis

Calories - 2000
Cholesterol - 80 mg
Protein - 95 g
Sodium - 1600 mg
Carbs - 285 g
Fiber - 40 g
Total fat - 48 g
Potassium - 3000 mg
Saturated fat - 4 g
Calcium - 1225 mg

Day 3 Sample

Breakfast

1 cup Red River Cereal with 1/2 cup berries
1/2 whole grain bagel
1 tsp soft margarine
1 cup sliced grapefruit/oranges
1/2 cup yogurt
Decaf coffee
Water

Lunch

Turkey lettuce wraps
  *1/2 cup sliced turkey
  *1/2 cup diced tomato
  *1/4 cup diced cucumber
  *1/4 cup shredded cheese
  *2 large Romaine lettuce leafs to fill
  *Drizzle mustard or mayo
2 cups steamed broccoli/carrots
Banana
Tea
Water

Dinner

3 ounce grilled tuna steak
1 cup cooked brown rice
1/2 grilled eggplant
1/2 grilled sweet potato
Orange Bubbly
  *3/4 cup fresh orange juice
  *1/4 cup sparkling water

Snack (anytime)

Mango
1 cup low-fat yogurt

Nutrition Analysis

Calories - 1900
Cholesterol - 100 mg
Protein - 100 g
Sodium - 900 mg
Carbs - 255 g
Fiber - 30 g
Total fat - 48 g
Potassium - 4500 mg
Saturated fat - 7 g
Calcium - 1200 mg

The Extras

When cooking your meals, don't add extra oils, butter, or fats. Pam works great in the pan, or you can add a drizzle of olive oil if you like. Just brush a tad on your meat when grilling, steam your veggies, and add herbs if you like, but you don't need to douse with salt and butter. All that does is mask the fantabulous flavors.

With rolls, buns, and bread, try them naked or with just a smear of margarine. Another alternative is a smear or jam or honey, or better yet peanut butter.

Steer clear of creamy sauces and condiments. If you've gotta have mayonnaise on your wrap, 1 tsp of low-fat is plenty. Sour cream doesn't need to sit atop your sweet potato. You can sprinkle a little thyme if you like, or perhaps a tbsp. of shredded cheese.

One manageable step at a time and you WILL get there!

My Thoughts...

Changing your eating strategy is tough. Heck, any sort of changes seems difficult. By focusing on creating new healthier eating habits with the DASH Diet, you'll slowly but surely zap your old unhealthy ways.

Don't focus on breaking habits, rather making new smart ones. Before you know it, you'll transform these new healthy eating changes into habit, your new normal, and it only gets better from there.

Chapter Nine - DASH Tips on the Run

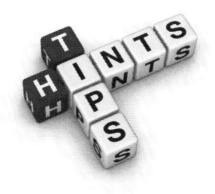

In order for your healthy new eating plan to stick, it's gotta fit in with your lifestyle. The reality is, most people end up eating on the run lots, out to restaurants and grabbing food during the day, when you're WAY past hungry.

By doing a little mental and physical prep work, you'll set yourself with the DASH Diet, to comfortable handle the eating situations you face when not on your home turf.

If you know you've got a busy week, try and pack extra snacks to curb your hunger, and deter you from hitting the closest fast food joint, or junky crap vending machine. Always carry a water bottle with you, so you're not grabbing soda. And if you need a little more, a diet pop is acceptable as a treat.

Healthy Snacks on the Go!

Cheese strings
Low-fat pudding
Veggie sticks
Yogurt
Boiled egg
1/2 cup raisins
1/4 cup mixed nuts
Banana
Apple
Pear
Orange
Whole grain cereal bar
Protein bar (careful on sugar)
1/4 cup dried fruit
1 cup mixed veggies
1/2 whole grain bread peanut butter sandwich with 1 tbsp. peanut butter
1/4 cup unsalted sunflower seeds
1/2 whole wheat bagel with 1 tbsp. light cream cheese
3/4 cup blueberries, strawberries, raspberries, or black-berries
1/2 grilled chicken breast

Just make sure you've got a few snacks in your car, office desk, or bag. When you're tired and hungry, emotions trump logic, and you don't want to go there.

PLANNING your food, is a fantabulous habit to get into!

EATING OUT TIP-TOP STRATEGIES FOR SUCCESS!

Easy on the Salt - Lowering your salt intake is one of your goals. Here are a few pointers to ponder when you're on strike from the kitchen:

*Remove the salt shaker off the table so you're not tempted to start shakin'!
*Ask the waiter to have your dishes prepared without salt, salt mixtures, or MSG.
*Use your noggin and don't order items you know are likely oozing with salt. Things like soups, dishes with soya sauce, or meats that are cured, have more salt than you need in a week!
*Back off the condiments high in salt. Like ketchup, barbecue sauce, relish, and mustard. A drizzle won't kill you anytime soon. But if you like to have a little bit of steak with your ketchup, you're going to have to smarten up!
*Don't be nibbling off other plates. Chances are the salt has already been added, and then some.

Call Ahead - If you know where you're going before, you can always ring the restaurant before you go with your list of questions. If you can figure out what you're going to order, and how you're going to order it beforehand, that gets rid of the guesswork. One less thing to worry about.

Be Wary of Unhealthy Fats - With the DASH Diet, you want to reduce fat and cholesterol. Here are a few tips to handle the fat when rippin' it up with a night on the town:

*Request low-fat salad dressing on the side.
*Ask that your dish be prepared without butter and extra oils.
*Choose lower fat dishes to start.
*Make sure your veggies are steamed naked - no salt or butter or dressing.
*Pick baked, broiled, steamed, grilled, poached, roasted, barbecued, or stir-fried WITHOUT oil.
*Cut visible fat off meat

Mind Over Matter with Portions - Restaurants suck when it comes to proper serving size. They typically serve 2-3 x's more than you need. Order a doggy bag BEFORE your meal arrives. Put half in before you take one bite. Right off the hop you've cut your usual fat and calorie intake in half.

Run from Appetizers - Unless you're having a naked house salad, you're best to skip the appetizers, especially the bread basket. Fried calamari, mozzarella sticks, creamy soups, nachos, egg rolls, and cheese stuffed anything, are all wrong.

You'll have plenty to eat with your healthy entree.

Say NO to dessert - If you have to have something sweet, opt for fresh fruit, low-fat rice pudding, sorbet, plain cake, or maybe baked apple. By no means, do you have to eat it all. A few bites, or sharing it with your bed buddy is a wise-owl move.

What's Best at Fast Food Joints - Even healthier fast food options can be dangerous. Most have the nutrition information readily available. Make sure you read it before ordering. If you've got to go junky, opt for the kid size burger and fries. And if you want to eat as healthy as possible, you should order the house salad with some *grilled* chicken, and a milk.

It's inevitable the chicken will likely be loaded with filler salt, but it's WAY better than a 1/4 pound greasy bacon double cheeseburger!

Pay Attention to the Menu - Many restaurants do a lot of the work for you, by placing cute little symbols beside dishes that are *heart healthy*, or *low in fat*. Have a look before ordering, and don't be afraid to ask questions.

74

Make a special request if you like. I've never run into a restaurant yet that isn't happy to accommodate.

DO NOT Finish Everything on your Plate - In order to find success in DASH eating, you've gotta learn to listen to your body, and stop eating before you're full. We're stuck in a world where emotion, habit, and boredom, drive crappy eating patterns. This bad eating is learned.

Guess what?

You can un-learn it!

Challenge yourself to leave some fuel on your plate. Little by little it's all going to add up.

My Thoughts...

Social pressures associated with eating are crazy dangerous. Learning to stand strong against them is going to help you take control of your eating, and turn your DASH Diet eating strategies into habit.

Set yourself up for success by focusing on the big picture. Be prepared when eating on the run, and pay attention to each and every good choice you make, down to the condiments.

Believe in yourself and it WILL happen!

Final Thoughts

The *NIH, National Institute of Health*, supported two research trials that clearly showed the benefits the DASH Diet eating concept had on decreasing blood pressure.

Think of this as the scientific tip of the mountain top. From there, it became evident the simple yet effective DASH Diet was so much more.

If Dr. Oz is on board, it's gotta be true!

Not to mention the fact, heath experts vote this eating strategy the BEST overall diet for the third year in a row.

There's no doubt the DASH Diet will help lower blood pressure, lose weight, deter disease, increase energy, stabilize your fat loss, increase motility and mobility, support quality sleep, reduce stress, and flip your life switch to positive.

The VIP question is whether or not you're willing to cut the crap and commit to it!

Unless you consciously decide you're ready to make healthy changes in your eating with this fantabulous eating strategy, it won't happen!

And if you're going to do it, you might as well do it right. Add to this regular intense interval weight and cardiovascular training, positive social relationships, friendships and romantic, along with finding the time you need to grow as a person. Where you make the time to discover new hobbies, take part in activities you love, and meditate, or maybe take a relaxing yoga session to de-stress.

Each of these factors are the basics you need to address to bring your health to optimal levels.

Stop talking about it.

Stop thinking about it.

The time has come for you to take positive action, full speed ahead, to a bright healthy future with the DASH Diet concept.

You deserve it!

Last Thoughts…

*THANK-YOU for reading my masterpiece. I hope you learned a little something, or at least got a few smiles.
*I would appreciate a millisecond or three of your time for a quick review, to help me build my masterful book empire higher.
*Whatever you do, don't forget to smile, and of course, check out my website for more of my e-Book masterpieces at: www.flawlesscreativewriting.com

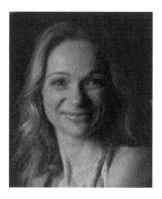

Cathy☺

Disclaimer

Manufactured by Amazon.ca
Bolton, ON

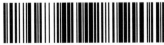